MORNING YOGA FOR SENIORS

Step by Step Guide to Strengthening Your Body and Mind in Just 10 minutes

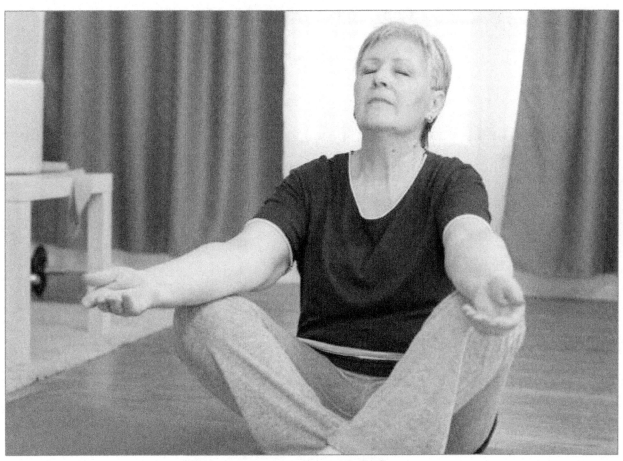

Dr. Laurie Miles

TABLE OF CONTENTS

INTRODUCTION

In the golden glow of a new day, as the world awakens, so too can your body and mind with the gentle embrace of Morning Yoga for Seniors. Imagine stepping onto a serene path of well-being, where just 10 minutes of dedicated practice can transform your mornings into moments of rejuvenation and strength.

Margaret, a spirited senior whose journey encapsulates the heart of this book. Struggling with the common challenges that come with age, she found herself yearning for vitality and a sense of connection. It was in the quiet hours of the morning that she discovered the transformative power of yoga. With each stretch and each breath, she felt her body slowly welcoming newfound flexibility and her mind embracing a sense of serenity.

Morning Yoga for Seniors is more than just a book; it's an empathetic guide crafted to enrich your life's chapters. If you've ever faced the stiffening grip of age, or the creeping doubts about your body's resilience, this book reaches out with understanding. It's a whisper of encouragement, reminding you that age is just a number, and the journey to wellness is yours to embark upon.

This guide is a roadmap to a healthier you. Within its pages, you'll find a carefully curated 10-minute yoga routine designed to gently awaken your body, strengthen your muscles, and nurture your mind. You'll explore the fundamental elements of yoga, learn how to adapt poses to your unique abilities, and uncover the powerful synergy between movement and mindfulness. More than just poses, this book is an invitation to cultivate a new connection with yourself — one that celebrates the beauty of aging gracefully.

Welcome to a journey of transformation, where each page invites you to rewrite your story. Let Morning Yoga for Seniors be your companion on this path, where the rising sun mirrors the awakening of your vitality. Your age is but a number, and your potential is boundless. With this guide, take the first step toward embracing a healthier, more vibrant you.

CHAPTER 1

Introduction to Morning Yoga

As the sun's first rays break through the dawn, a world of possibility awakens. In those tranquil moments, an opportunity to nourish both body and mind awaits – an opportunity found in the embrace of Morning Yoga for Seniors. Picture this: a simple practice that takes only 10 minutes, yet has the power to shape the rest of your day, infusing it with vitality and serenity.

<u>The Benefits of Morning Yoga for Seniors</u>

Age is but a chapter in the story of life, and every chapter deserves a touch of grace and renewal. Morning yoga, specifically tailored for seniors, holds a treasure trove of benefits that can make your golden years truly shine. Imagine greeting each day with increased flexibility, improved balance, and a heightened sense of well-being. These are not merely lofty promises; they are the tangible gifts that yoga bestows upon those who embrace its practice.

As the body ages, it can gradually lose its suppleness and strength. Joints may stiffen, muscles might weaken, and a general feeling of lethargy can set in. This is where morning yoga comes to your aid. Through gentle stretches, intentional movements, and mindful breathing, you can rejuvenate your body's systems, inviting a renewed sense of agility and ease. The postures and poses within your 10-minute practice are designed to enhance blood circulation, stimulate digestion, and promote joint mobility – a symphony of benefits that will set a harmonious tone for the day ahead.

Yet, the rewards of morning yoga extend far beyond the physical realm. Yoga is a holistic practice that weaves a tapestry of connections between the body, mind, and spirit. As you flow through your practice, you cultivate mindfulness, turning your attention inward to the present moment. The gentle guidance of your breath becomes a bridge to tranquility, as stress and worries gently dissipate. Studies have shown that a regular yoga practice can help lower blood pressure, reduce anxiety, and enhance overall mental clarity. It's not just about poses; it's about finding solace in the space between them.

How This Book Can Help You

This book is more than pages and words; it's a guiding light on your journey to well-being. If you've ever yearned for a way to start your day with intention, to embrace your age gracefully, and to foster a connection with yourself that transcends time, then this book is your companion.

Within these chapters, you'll find a wealth of knowledge carefully curated to cater to seniors looking to embark on a rejuvenating journey. We understand the unique challenges that come with age, and we acknowledge the need for practices that are both effective and accessible. That's why this book is a testament to empathy and inclusivity. Whether you're an experienced yogi or new to the mat, our step-by-step guide will meet you where you are, gently guiding you through each pose, each movement, and each breath.

In the upcoming pages, you'll be introduced to the foundational principles of yoga and its specific benefits for seniors. You'll learn how to create a sacred space for your practice, how to adapt poses to your body's abilities, and how to infuse mindfulness into your daily routine. Your 10-minute morning yoga practice will become a source of nourishment, not just for your body, but for your mind and spirit as well.

As you delve into the heart of this book, remember that it's not about achieving perfection; it's about embracing progress. It's about cherishing every small victory, celebrating each moment of self-care, and savoring the joy that comes from moving your body and quieting your mind. You deserve a life that's brimming with vitality and wellness, and this book is here to guide you toward that life.

So, as we embark on this journey together, let's welcome the mornings with open arms, inviting the power of yoga to shape our days, one breath, one pose, and one sunrise at a time. Your age is a testament to the richness of your experiences, and your practice will become a testament to your dedication to self-care and well-being. The path is laid out before you – are you ready to take the first step?

CHAPTER 2

Understanding the Basics of Yoga

In the realm of wellness and self-discovery, yoga stands as a beacon of ancient wisdom, offering a transformative journey that transcends time and age. As we dive into the foundations of yoga, let's explore the essence of this practice, understand why it's a perfect fit for seniors, and delve into the importance of safety considerations.

<u>What is Yoga?</u>

Yoga, a Sanskrit word that translates to "union" or "to yoke," encapsulates a holistic approach to connecting the mind, body, and spirit. At its core, yoga is not merely a set of physical postures, but a philosophy that guides individuals toward a state of balance and harmony. Rooted in the teachings of ancient India, yoga was originally developed as a path to self-realization and enlightenment. Over time, it has evolved into a multifaceted practice that spans physical, mental, and spiritual dimensions.

Central to yoga is the concept of mindfulness, a state of heightened awareness that directs our attention to the present moment. Through conscious breathing and intentional movement, practitioners cultivate mindfulness, allowing them to step away from the distractions of daily life and immerse themselves in the richness of the here and now. It's a practice that encourages self-reflection, self-acceptance, and the cultivation of inner peace.

Why Yoga is Suitable for Seniors

Age is not a barrier to embarking on a transformative journey of well-being; rather, it's an invitation to explore new avenues of self-care and growth. Yoga, with its gentle yet profound approach, is perfectly suited for seniors who seek to enhance their quality of life and embrace the golden years with grace.

The beauty of yoga lies in its adaptability. Each pose can be modified to cater to various levels of flexibility and strength. This inherent flexibility makes yoga an inclusive practice, accommodating individuals with diverse abilities. Seniors, often navigating the changes that come with age, can find solace in knowing that yoga meets them where they are.

Yoga's benefits for seniors are manifold. The gentle stretches and movements foster joint mobility and muscle strength, counteracting the stiffness that can accompany aging. As balance becomes a focus, standing and balancing poses promote stability, reducing the risk of falls. Furthermore, yoga's mindful nature supports cognitive well-being, enhancing mental clarity and reducing stress – a gift that resonates deeply as life's pace slows down.

Safety Considerations

While yoga holds a wealth of benefits, it's essential to prioritize safety, particularly for seniors. Each body is unique, and understanding your body's limitations is crucial to a safe and fulfilling practice. Before embarking on your yoga journey, consult with your healthcare provider to ensure that yoga aligns with your health status and any medical considerations.

As you explore yoga poses, listen to your body's signals. Gentle discomfort is normal as you stretch and move, but pain is not. Avoid pushing yourself into positions that feel painful or straining. Instead, focus on gradual progression, allowing your body to adapt and grow at its own pace.

Props, such as blocks, straps, and bolsters, are invaluable tools that offer support and stability. They can aid in achieving proper alignment and reduce the risk of overexertion. Utilizing props is a testament to the wisdom of adapting your practice to suit your body's unique needs.

In conclusion, understanding the essence of yoga, its suitability for seniors, and the importance of safety considerations sets the stage for a fulfilling journey of self-discovery and well-being. As you venture into the world of yoga, remember that this practice is a gift you give to yourself – a gift of movement, mindfulness, and connection. With each breath, you forge a path toward vitality and self-care, embracing the chapters of life with strength and grace.

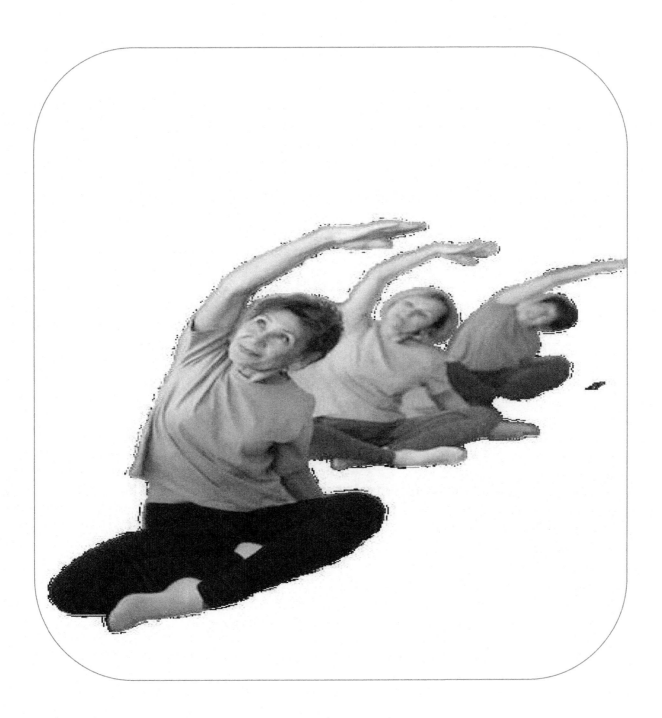

CHAPTER 3

Getting Started with Your Practice

Embarking on a journey of self-care through morning yoga is akin to stepping into a sacred sanctuary, where your body and mind find solace and renewal. As we begin our exploration of the essentials, let's delve into the art of setting up your practice space, understanding the necessary equipment, and immersing ourselves in the gentle embrace of breathing techniques for relaxation.

<u>Setting Up Your Space</u>

Your practice space is more than just a physical location; it's a reflection of your commitment to well-being. Selecting the right space can significantly enhance your experience, creating an environment that encourages focus, tranquility, and mindfulness.

Ideally, choose a quiet and clutter-free area that allows you to move freely without hindrance. Natural light can infuse the space with a sense of vitality, but if that's not available, opt for soft, warm lighting that fosters a serene ambiance. If possible, dedicate a corner or a portion of a room solely to your practice, creating a sense of ritual and intention.

Decorate your space with elements that resonate with you – perhaps a soothing painting, a Himalayan salt lamp, or a few potted plants. A touch of nature can amplify the sense of connection with the world around you. Lay down a comfortable mat that supports your body as you move through poses. And finally, consider having a small table or shelf nearby to hold any props or accessories you might need.

Necessary Equipment

Yoga's beauty lies in its simplicity, requiring minimal equipment to embark on your journey. The essentials are designed to support and enhance your practice, allowing you to fully immerse yourself in the experience.

Yoga Mat: A high-quality yoga mat provides cushioning and traction, ensuring your safety and comfort as you transition between poses.

Props: Depending on your needs, props such as blocks, straps, and bolsters can aid in achieving proper alignment and support. They're especially beneficial for seniors looking to adapt poses to their abilities.

Comfortable Attire: Wear clothing that allows you to move freely and comfortably. Choose breathable fabrics that enable your skin to breathe, facilitating an enjoyable practice.

Water Bottle: Staying hydrated is essential, even during a gentle yoga practice. Keep a water bottle nearby to ensure you can take sips as needed.

Blanket or Towel: Having a blanket or towel nearby can provide warmth and support during seated or lying poses.

Breathing Techniques for Relaxation

Breath is the thread that weaves together every aspect of your yoga practice. Learning to harness the power of your breath can transform your practice from a series of physical movements to a profound journey of mindfulness and relaxation.

Begin with Diaphragmatic breathing: Find a comfortable seated position. Close your eyes and place one hand on your chest and the other on your abdomen. Take a long, slow breath in through your nose, feeling your belly rise as your lungs fill with air. Exhale slowly, feeling your abdomen fall. This technique calms the nervous system and centers your focus on your breath.

Alternate Nostril Breathing: This technique balances the left and right hemispheres of the brain, promoting mental clarity and relaxation. Using your right thumb, close off your right nostril and inhale through your left nostril. At the top of the inhale, close off your left nostril with your right ring finger and release your right nostril. Exhale through your right nostril. Inhale through your right nostril, then close it off and exhale through your left nostril. Practice this breathing exercise for a few rounds.

Ujjayi Breath: Also known as "Victorious Breath," Ujjayi breath involves a gentle constriction at the back of the throat. Inhale slowly through your nose, and as you exhale, create a gentle hissing sound in the back of your throat. This technique calms the mind and supports focus during your practice.

As you embark on your morning yoga journey, remember that your breath is your constant companion, guiding you through each movement and helping you cultivate a sense of presence and tranquility. With the foundation of your practice space, the essential equipment, and the power of conscious breathing, you're well on your way to creating a haven of well-being that honors both your body and your mind.

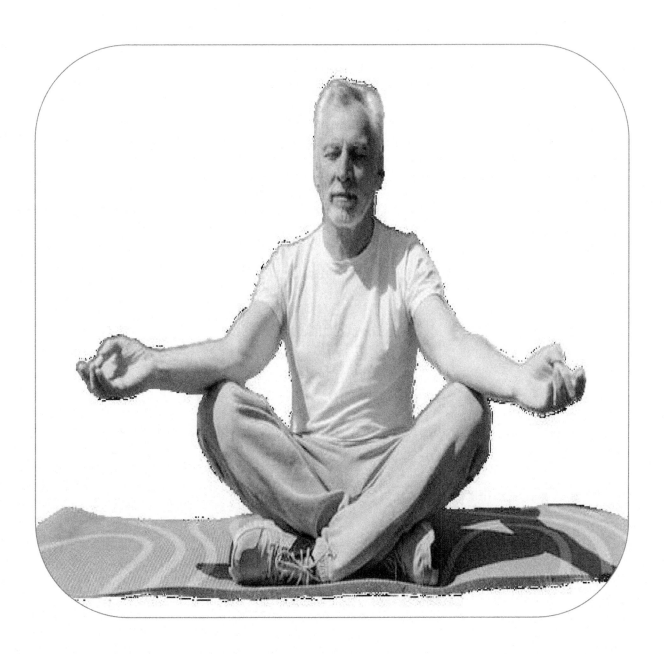

CHAPTER 4

10-Minute Morning Yoga Routine

Embark on a journey of revitalization that unfolds in just 10 minutes. Within this brief yet profound window of time, you have the opportunity to nurture your body, calm your mind, and set a positive trajectory for the day. This carefully curated morning yoga routine is designed to weave together movement, mindfulness, and breath, creating a symphony of well-being that resonates throughout your being. Let's take this journey one step at a time and see where it takes us.

Gentle Warm-Up Exercises

As the sun's early rays grace the horizon, begin your morning yoga routine with a series of gentle warm-up exercises. These preliminary movements serve as a heartfelt welcome to your body, gradually awakening your muscles, joints, and senses. Consider this the tender embrace you offer to yourself, preparing your physical vessel for the transformative practice that lies ahead.

Neck Stretches: Gently tilt your head from side to side, inviting a gentle release of tension that might have accrued during your restful slumber.

Shoulder Rolls: Envision rolling away any burdens or worries as you rotate your shoulders forward and backward. Feel the gentle unwinding of knots and stiffness.

Wrist and Ankle Circles: In these simple circular motions, find a connection to the rhythmic pulse of your body. Through the movements of your extremities, you establish a connection with the core of your being.

Cat-Cow Stretch: As you transition into the cat-cow sequence, create a dialogue between your spine and breath. Inhale, arching your back like a contented cat, and exhale, rounding your spine like a gentle cow.

With each movement, with each breath, you lay the foundation for a practice that honors the interconnectedness of your body's elements.

Sun Salutations for Seniors

Modified sun salutations form the heart of your morning yoga routine. These graceful movements, imbued with intention, mimic the progression of the sun as it climbs higher into the sky, casting its warm glow upon the world. As you flow through this sequence, visualize the dawn of possibility, the emergence of vitality, and the embrace of serenity.

Mountain Pose: Root yourself to the ground, feeling the strength and stability of the earth beneath you. Inhale as you raise your arms overhead, fingertips reaching for the heavens. Imagine yourself as a sturdy mountain, unwavering in your presence.

Forward Fold: Exhale gracefully, folding forward from your hips. In this forward fold, surrender any remnants of stiffness or resistance, allowing your body to cascade like a waterfall toward the ground.

Half Forward Fold: Inhale and find a midway point, lengthening your spine. Imagine your body as a bridge, connecting the earth below with the sky above.

Modified Low Plank: As you step or ease your way back into a modified low plank position, you embrace strength and humility. Here, your body becomes a canvas upon which determination is painted.

Cobra or Upward-Facing Dog: Inhale, lifting your chest as you enter cobra or a gentler version of upward-facing dog. Feel your heart expanding, greeting the morning light.

Downward-Facing Dog: Exhale, transitioning into downward-facing dog. In this inverted pose, visualize yourself as a pyramid connecting heaven and earth, as your body radiates energy and purpose.

Half Forward Fold: Inhale, returning to the halfway point, bridging the gap between the earth and sky.

Forward Fold: Exhale and fold forward once again, a fluid movement that mirrors the passage of time and the continuous cycle of renewal.

Mountain Pose: Inhale deeply, rising gracefully to mountain pose. As you stretch your arms overhead, embrace the potential of a new day, open and full of promise.

Standing and Balancing Poses

Standing poses embody a sense of rootedness, while balancing poses challenge your stability, both physically and metaphorically. In these moments of equilibrium, you cultivate a connection between your body's foundation and your aspirations.

Tree Pose: Root one foot into the ground while bringing the sole of the other foot to your calf or thigh. Extend your arms toward the heavens, like branches seeking the sky. Find a focal point, an anchor, as you balance.

Warrior II: Step back into warrior II, where strength and grace intertwine. As you extend your arms and gaze over your front hand, feel the expansiveness of your stance and the unwavering spirit within you.

With each pose, a dialogue unfolds between your physical presence and the realm of possibilities that stretches before you.

Seated and Floor Poses

Transitioning into seated and floor poses provides a grounding experience, inviting a sense of introspection and calmness. Here, the world outside fades, and your inner world takes center stage.

Seated Forward Fold: As you ease into a seated forward fold, your body gently unfurls like a blossoming flower. Your spine elongates, and with each breath, you release tensions that may have gathered during the night.

Butterfly Pose: In butterfly pose, the soles of your feet come together, a symbol of unity. Your knees fall gently to the sides, embracing openness. With each breath, imagine yourself as a butterfly, ready to take flight into a day filled with possibilities.

Final Relaxation and Mindfulness

As your practice winds down, you find yourself in a space of tranquility and quietude. The final poses offer you an opportunity to integrate the movements, sensations, and emotions that have coursed through your being.

Corpse Pose (Savasana): In savasana, you lie down, arms by your sides, palms facing upward. This pose mirrors the stillness of the earth at dawn, as you surrender into the embrace of your mat. Close your eyes, inviting a deep sense of restfulness.

Mindfulness Meditation: As you lie in savasana, your breath becomes your anchor. Inhale deeply through your nose, allowing the air to fill your lungs. Exhale gently, releasing any residual tension. With each breath, create space within yourself, where tranquility and clarity flourish.

With the timer marking the completion of your 10-minute morning yoga routine, take a moment to acknowledge the harmony you've cultivated within yourself. Through the choreography of movement, breath, and mindfulness, you've woven a tapestry of well-being that will accompany you throughout the day.

Remember that this practice is a reflection of your commitment to nurturing your body and tending to your spirit. With each pose, each breath, you've created a sacred space where vitality and serenity converge. Carry this sense of centeredness with you as you step into the day, knowing that within you lies a reservoir of strength, balance, and tranquility. The sun has risen, and so have you, awakening to a day brimming with potential and promise.

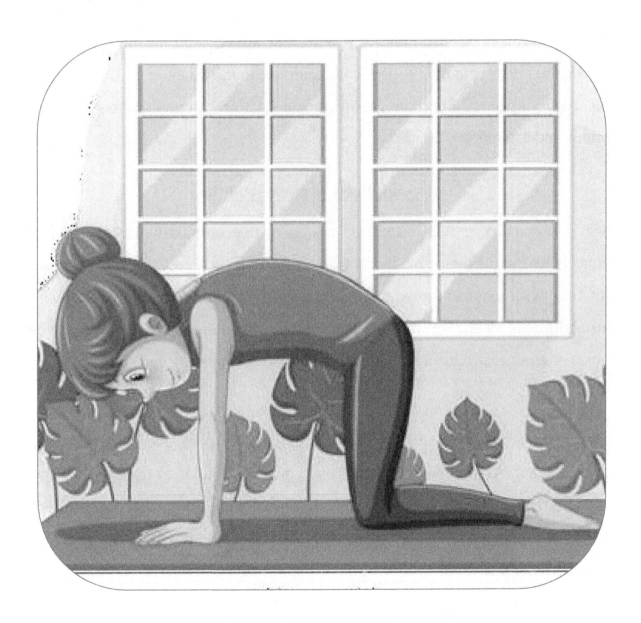

CHAPTER 5

Modifying Poses for Seniors

In the realm of yoga, the mat becomes a canvas for self-expression, and each pose is an opportunity to cultivate a deep connection with your body. As a senior practitioner, you bring a lifetime of experiences and wisdom to the mat, and it's important to honor your unique needs and abilities. In this chapter, we delve into the art of modifying poses for seniors, allowing you to tailor your practice to your body's rhythms and aspirations.

Adapting Poses to Your Abilities

Yoga is a practice of self-awareness, a journey that unfolds within your body's unique landscape. Embracing the concept of modifying poses is not a sign of limitation; it's a testament to your wisdom and self-compassion. Adapting poses to your abilities is an empowering act that allows you to engage with yoga on your terms, fostering a sustainable practice that nourishes both body and spirit.

Listen to Your Body: Your body is a repository of wisdom, and its signals guide you on the mat. As you move through poses, pay close attention to how your body responds. If a pose feels uncomfortable or causes pain, honor that feedback and modify accordingly. Remember, your practice is a dialogue with your body, and every adjustment you make reflects your commitment to self-care.

Explore Gentle Variations: Yoga is not a competition; it's a personal journey of growth and self-discovery. Embrace gentle variations of poses that resonate with your current abilities. For instance, if a traditional plank pose is challenging, consider modifying it by lowering your knees to the ground, maintaining the core engagement without strain.

Use Props Mindfully: Props are your allies in the realm of modification. Blocks, straps, bolsters, and blankets can provide invaluable support, enhancing your practice's accessibility and comfort. For instance, if you struggle with balance in standing poses, a chair can offer stability. Utilizing props allows you to experience the essence of a pose without compromising your well-being.

Using Props for Support

Props are the silent heroes of your yoga practice, offering a bridge between where you are and where you aspire to be. They create a safe and nurturing environment that invites exploration and growth. By integrating props into your practice, you weave a tapestry of support that acknowledges your body's present state while fostering a journey of expansion.

Blocks: Blocks are versatile tools that provide stability and extension. They can elevate the floor to meet your body, offering a sense of accessibility in poses like forward folds or triangle poses. By using blocks mindfully, you ensure that your body's alignment remains intact, preventing strain and promoting comfort.

Straps: Straps offer an extended reach, enabling you to engage with poses that demand flexibility beyond your current range. For example, in seated forward folds, a strap can act as an extension of your arms, allowing you to explore the pose with ease. Straps empower you to experience the fullness of a pose without compromising your body's integrity.

Bolsters and Pillows: Bolsters and pillows invite a sense of relaxation and restoration into your practice. They create a sanctuary of comfort, allowing you to sink into restorative poses with grace. Placing a bolster under your knees in savasana (corpse pose) or using pillows to support your body in gentle backbends ensures that your practice becomes a haven of self-care.

Blankets: Blankets provide both comfort and warmth, enhancing your practice's nurturing essence. Rolling up a blanket to place under your knees in kneeling poses or using it as a cushion for seated poses brings a sense of cushioning to your practice. Blankets adapt to your body's needs, ensuring that each pose is an experience of gentle support.

As you navigate the journey of modifying poses for seniors, remember that each modification is a celebration of your body's resilience and a testament to your dedication to self-care. Yoga is a journey of self-discovery, and by adapting poses to your abilities and embracing the support of props, you're embarking on a path of mindful movement that reflects your unique essence. Your practice is a canvas upon which you paint a masterpiece of self-expression and vitality. With each modification, each exploration, you're crafting a practice that honors your body's wisdom and nurtures your spirit's aspirations. Through mindful modification, you're creating a practice that resonates with the rhythms of your body and empowers you to journey through life with grace and strength.

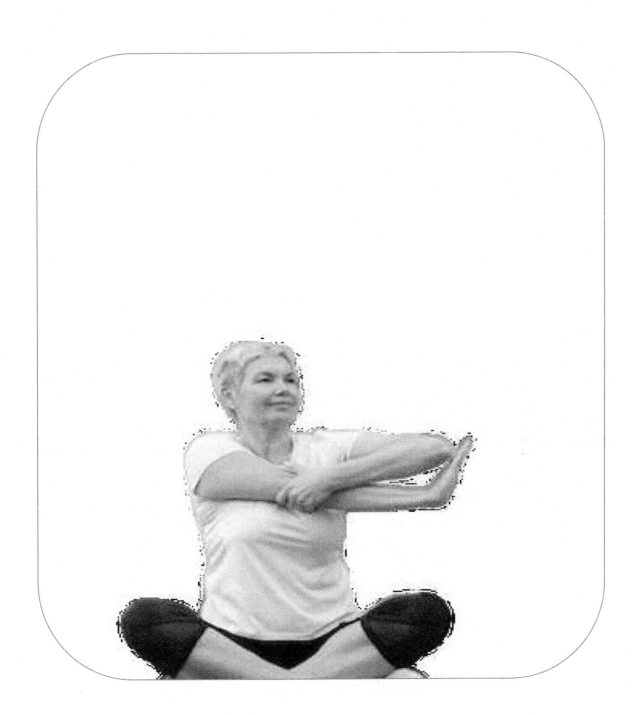

CHAPTER 6

Overcoming Common Challenges

In the journey of life, challenges often become stepping stones to growth. The same principle applies to your yoga practice. As a senior practitioner, you bring a unique tapestry of experiences to your mat, and with it, you may encounter certain challenges. In this chapter, we delve into overcoming common challenges, embracing them as opportunities to deepen your practice, foster resilience, and cultivate a profound connection with your body and mind.

Dealing with Stiffness and Soreness

Stiffness and soreness are natural companions of aging, reminders of a life well-lived. However, they need not be barriers to a vibrant yoga practice. In fact, yoga can be a soothing balm that eases these discomforts, provided you approach it with mindfulness and self-compassion.

Mindful Movement: Embrace the philosophy of "gentle is the new advanced." Begin your practice with mindful movements that gradually awaken your muscles and joints. Slow, deliberate stretches and gentle rotations can alleviate stiffness and initiate a gentle dialogue with your body.

Dynamic Warm-Ups: Engage in dynamic warm-up sequences that coax your body out of its slumber. Incorporate movements like neck rolls, shoulder circles, and ankle rotations to infuse your body with warmth and vitality.

Breath Awareness: Your breath is a bridge between your body and mind. As you move through poses, focus on deep, intentional breathing. Inhale to create space, exhale to release tension. The rhythm of your breath serves as a gentle massage, soothing your muscles and inviting suppleness.

Hydration and Nutrition: Adequate hydration and balanced nutrition play a pivotal role in managing stiffness and soreness. Water keeps your joints lubricated, and a diet rich in anti-inflammatory foods like fruits, vegetables, and omega-3 fatty acids can alleviate discomfort.

Managing Limited Mobility

Limited mobility doesn't signify limitation of potential. Instead, it prompts creative exploration and an invitation to redefine movement within your own parameters. Yoga is a practice of adaptation, and through modifications and patience, you can embrace a practice that honors your body's unique capabilities.

Celebrate Small Victories: Each movement, no matter how subtle, is a victory. Celebrate the range of motion you have, and let it be a source of motivation. With time, consistent practice may yield surprising improvements.

Adapt Poses: Modification is not a sign of weakness; it's a testament to your wisdom. Adjust poses to suit your mobility. If a full pose isn't attainable, find a variation that allows you to engage and experience the essence of the pose.

Prop-Assisted Poses: Props are your allies in expanding your practice's horizons. For instance, a chair can provide support in seated poses or balance-challenging poses. Use blocks to bridge the gap between your body and the floor, allowing you to explore poses with comfort.

Mindset Shift: Embrace a mindset of curiosity rather than frustration. Approach your practice as an exploration, where each movement holds the potential for discovery. With each attempt, you're redefining movement and creating a canvas of possibility.

Finding Motivation and Consistency

In the tapestry of life, motivation and consistency are threads that weave a vibrant pattern of growth. Yet, it's normal to encounter periods where these threads waver. Rediscovering motivation and nurturing consistency is a gentle dance that requires self-kindness and intention.

Set Realistic Goals: Set achievable goals that reflect your current abilities and aspirations. These goals act as guideposts, illuminating your path and fostering a sense of purpose.

Create Rituals: Establish a daily routine that carves out time for your practice. Whether it's a dedicated morning slot or a peaceful evening ritual, these moments of self-care become anchors that keep you connected to your practice.

Variety and Curiosity: Introduce variety into your practice to keep it engaging. Experiment with different styles of yoga, explore new poses, and embrace a spirit of curiosity. Variety breathes life into your practice, infusing it with freshness and excitement.

Mindful Progress Tracking: Document your journey as a testament to your growth. Note how you feel after each practice, the poses you've explored, and the sensations in your body. These records become a wellspring of motivation and a testament to your progress.

CHAPTER 7

Enhancing Your Mind-Body Connection

The journey of yoga is a multi-dimensional exploration that extends beyond the physical postures and movements. As a senior practitioner, you have the unique opportunity to deepen your mind-body connection, fostering a harmonious relationship between your physical self and your inner world. In this chapter, we will delve into the transformative power of mindfulness and the profound impact that yoga can have on your mental well-being.

Incorporating Mindfulness into Your Practice

Mindfulness is the art of paying attention to what is happening now, without judgment. It's a conscious awareness of your thoughts, feelings, bodily sensations, and the environment around you. Integrating mindfulness into your yoga practice enriches each movement and breath, creating a meditative flow that not only enhances your physical practice but also nurtures your mental and emotional well-being.

The Breath as Your Anchor: Begin your practice by drawing your attention to your breath. With each inhalation and exhalation, observe the natural rhythm of your breath. This simple act of awareness serves as an anchor, grounding you in the present moment and helping you transcend distractions.

Embodiment through Body Scan: Progress through your practice with a mindful body scan. As you move through each pose, direct your attention to the sensations in various parts of your body. This practice cultivates a profound awareness of your body's responses and invites a gentle dialogue with its needs.

Savoring Each Moment: Instead of rushing through poses to check them off your list, savor each moment within a pose. As you transition from one pose to another, immerse yourself fully in the experience. Feel the stretch, notice the engagement of muscles, and follow the ebb and flow of your breath.

Witnessing Thoughts: Your mind may wander during your practice, and that's completely natural. When thoughts arise, acknowledge them without judgment, and then gently guide your focus back to your breath or the sensations of the pose. This process of releasing thoughts and returning to the present moment is a fundamental aspect of mindfulness.

Cultivating Gratitude: Dedicate a few moments before or after your practice to cultivating gratitude. Reflect on the gift of your body's abilities, the space you have to practice, and the opportunity to engage with yoga. This practice shifts your perspective, fostering a sense of contentment and presence.

Yoga's Impact on Mental Well-Being

While yoga is often associated with physical flexibility and strength, its impact extends far beyond the body. As a senior practitioner, you are poised to experience the profound effects of yoga on your mental and emotional well-being, enriching your inner landscape and fostering resilience.

Stress Reduction: The complexities of modern life can lead to the accumulation of stress. Yoga provides a sanctuary where you can release stress and tension. By synchronizing movement and breath, you activate the body's relaxation response, soothing the nervous system and inviting a sense of calm.

Mind-Body Harmony: Yoga encourages a symbiotic relationship between your body and mind. Mindful engagement with poses enhances your ability to listen to your body's cues, promoting self-awareness and self-compassion. The result is a harmonious coexistence that extends into your daily life.

Emotional Regulation: Yoga offers a safe space to explore and release emotions. As you navigate poses, emotions may rise to the surface. Rather than suppressing them, observe them with compassion. Over time, this practice of emotional exploration fosters emotional intelligence and resilience.

Cultivating Presence: The heart of yoga lies in its emphasis on presence. By cultivating mindfulness during your practice, you sharpen your ability to be fully engaged in each moment. This heightened presence translates beyond the mat, fostering a sense of centeredness and clarity in your daily activities.

Nurturing Patience: The journey of yoga is patient and gradual, emphasizing progress over perfection. This cultivation of patience within your practice has a ripple effect in your everyday life, enabling you to navigate challenges with grace and equanimity.

Prioritizing Self-Care: Consistent engagement in a yoga practice is an act of profound self-care. It sends a powerful message that your well-being matters. This nurturing ritual enhances your sense of self-worth and empowers you to prioritize your needs.

Yoga's impact on mental well-being is a testament to its holistic nature. It acknowledges that you are not just a physical body but a complex tapestry of thoughts, emotions, and experiences. As you continue to delve into your practice, remember that yoga is a journey of integration – a dance that unites your physical, mental, and spiritual dimensions. By infusing mindfulness into your practice and embracing yoga's impact on your mental well-being, you're embarking on a transformative path that has the potential to enrich your life beyond measure. With each mindful breath and intentional movement, you're fostering a profound connection between your mind and body, nurturing a state of harmony that resonates throughout your life journey.

CHAPTER 8

Tips for Long-Term Progress

In the realm of yoga, progress is a tapestry woven through consistent practice, patience, and a willingness to explore. As a senior practitioner, your journey is enriched by years of wisdom and experience. In this chapter, we delve into valuable tips for fostering long-term progress in your practice, ensuring that your journey is one of continual growth, self-discovery, and vibrant well-being.

Tracking Your Progress

The path of progress is illuminated by the light of awareness. Tracking your journey allows you to celebrate milestones, acknowledge growth, and make informed decisions about your practice. Embrace these strategies to keep a mindful record of your evolution.

Journaling Your Practice: Maintain a practice journal where you record your experiences, thoughts, and reflections after each session. Note the poses you explored, any challenges you faced, and moments of breakthrough. This journal becomes a personal repository of your journey, offering insight into your progress.

Photographic Documentation: Periodically take photos of your practice. These visual snapshots provide a tangible reflection of your growth. As you compare photos over time, you'll witness the subtle shifts in alignment, flexibility, and strength.

Creating a Progress Chart: Develop a chart that outlines your goals, both short-term and long-term. As you practice, mark your achievements, no matter how small. This visual representation of your progress can be a powerful motivator.

Celebrate Micro-Progress: Sometimes progress isn't monumental; it's found in the minutiae. Celebrate each small step forward, whether it's holding a pose for a few seconds longer or experiencing a newfound sense of ease in a challenging pose.

Gradually Increasing Intensity

Progress is a patient journey that flourishes through incremental steps. By gradually increasing the intensity of your practice, you cultivate a foundation of strength, flexibility, and endurance that can withstand the test of time.

Practicing Mindful Progression: Approach your practice with an attitude of mindful progression. If a particular pose feels accessible, gently explore variations that add depth. Progressing with mindfulness prevents injury and encourages sustainable growth.

Adding Repetition: As you become comfortable with certain poses, consider adding repetitions. This approach not only enhances your endurance but also deepens your understanding of the pose's nuances.

Exploring Balancing Poses: Balancing poses offer a unique challenge that engages both body and mind. As you explore poses like tree pose or warrior III, you cultivate stability and focus, contributing to your overall progress.

Utilizing Dynamic Movements: Integrate dynamic movements into your practice, such as dynamic lunges, gentle twists, or controlled transitions. These movements engage different muscle groups, fostering a well-rounded practice.

Incorporating Variety

Variety is the spice that keeps your practice vibrant and engaging. By incorporating diverse elements, you not only prevent monotony but also stimulate your body's capacity to adapt and evolve.

Exploring Different Styles: Yoga is a rich tapestry with a myriad of styles to explore. Venture beyond your comfort zone by experimenting with styles like restorative, Yin, or Vinyasa. Each style brings a unique perspective to your practice.

Sampling New Poses: The yoga landscape is brimming with poses waiting to be discovered. Dedicate a portion of your practice to exploring new poses. Each pose you introduce challenges your body in fresh ways, contributing to your growth.

Embracing Prop Utilization: Props are your companions on the journey of variety. Incorporating props like blocks, straps, and blankets opens doors to new variations and expressions of poses.

Mindful Sequencing: Design your practice with thoughtful sequencing that balances different types of poses. Pair strength-building poses with gentle stretches, ensuring a well-rounded practice that engages your body holistically.

Fostering long-term progress in your yoga practice is a testament to your commitment to self-care and personal growth. Through tracking your journey, gradually increasing intensity, and incorporating variety, you cultivate a practice that adapts to your evolving needs. Each pose, each breath, and each moment on your mat become a celebration of your journey – a journey of resilience, curiosity, and a profound connection with your body, mind, and spirit.

Chapter 9

Incorporating Yoga into Your Daily Life

Yoga is a timeless practice that extends far beyond the confines of a yoga mat. It's a way of living that can infuse each day with mindfulness, vitality, and a deep sense of well-being. As a senior practitioner, integrating yoga into your daily routine holds the potential to transform how you experience the world around you. In this chapter, we delve into the art of seamlessly weaving yoga into various aspects of your daily life, cultivating a harmonious connection between your practice and your existence.

Beyond the Morning Routine

While starting your day with a dedicated morning yoga routine is a wonderful practice, the spirit of yoga can accompany you throughout your entire day. Embrace these strategies to infuse your daily activities with the essence of yoga:

Mindful Breath: Yoga is deeply intertwined with conscious breathing. Take a few deep breaths throughout the day to center yourself and bring yourself back to the present moment. This simple practice can be especially helpful during moments of stress or when you're seeking clarity.

Mindful Eating: Approach each meal with mindfulness and gratitude. Before you begin eating, take a moment to appreciate the nourishment in front of you. As you eat, savor each bite, paying attention to the flavors, textures, and sensations as they unfold.

Desk Yoga: If you find yourself spending extended periods at a desk, integrate mini yoga sessions into your routine. Engage in gentle stretches, seated twists, and wrist circles to alleviate tension and invigorate your body and mind.

Walking Meditation: Transform your daily walk into a walking meditation. As you stroll, direct your attention to your breath and the sensation of your feet touching the ground. This practice keeps you active while nurturing a heightened sense of mindfulness.

Joining Senior Yoga Classes

Engaging in yoga classes specifically tailored for seniors offers an inclusive and supportive environment in which you can thrive and learn alongside peers who share similar life experiences. These classes not only deepen your practice but also nurture a sense of community:

Tailored Practices: Senior yoga classes are meticulously designed to cater to your unique needs. Instructors offer modifications and variations that respect your body's capabilities, ensuring a safe and effective practice.

Community Connection: Joining a senior yoga class creates a sense of belonging and camaraderie. You're surrounded by individuals who understand the nuances of aging and can provide a supportive network for your journey.

Guidance from Experts: Instructors of senior yoga classes possess the expertise to adapt poses and sequences to suit your specific requirements. Their knowledge ensures that you experience the benefits of yoga while avoiding any potential strain or injury.

Accountability and Consistency: Attending regular classes adds an element of accountability to your practice. The structured environment of a class encourages you to maintain a consistent practice, leading to improved well-being.

Yoga Retreats and Community

Yoga retreats and community events offer immersive experiences that take your practice to new depths and cultivate meaningful connections with fellow practitioners. These gatherings provide an opportunity to enrich your journey and explore yoga on a more profound level:

Retreats for Rejuvenation: Consider participating in yoga retreats designed specifically for seniors. Often held in serene settings, these retreats allow you to disconnect from your daily routine and immerse yourself in intensive practice and self-care.

Learning from Experts: Retreats typically feature expert instructors who lead sessions delving into yoga philosophy, meditation, and breath work. Exposure to these teachings broadens your perspective and deepens your practice.

Cultivating Connections: Yoga retreats and community events provide a platform to connect with like-minded individuals who share your passion for well-being. These connections can extend beyond the event, enriching your daily life with shared experiences.

Holistic Experience: Beyond the physical asana practice, retreats often include sessions on nutrition, wellness, and mindfulness. This holistic approach equips you with tools to enhance various facets of your life, ensuring a comprehensive and transformative experience.

Incorporating yoga into your daily life transcends the physical practice; it's an invitation to embody yoga's philosophy and principles in every moment. Beyond your morning routine, you have the opportunity to infuse mindfulness into your actions, join senior yoga classes for tailored guidance and a sense of community, and explore the transformative experiences offered by yoga retreats and community events.

Chapter 10

Frequently Asked Questions

Embarking on a yoga journey as a senior practitioner often brings forth questions and uncertainties. In this section, we address common concerns and misconceptions to provide you with a comprehensive understanding of how yoga can enrich your life.

Addressing Common Concerns

Is yoga suitable for seniors with limited mobility?

Absolutely. Yoga's beauty lies in its adaptability. Seniors with limited mobility can engage in a yoga practice tailored to their needs. Certified instructors are skilled at modifying poses, making them accessible and beneficial. These modifications respect your unique abilities while fostering progress.

Moreover, gentle yoga styles like Yin and Restorative yoga are particularly accommodating for seniors seeking to enhance flexibility, mobility, and overall well-being. These practices involve longer holds of poses and focus on relaxation and stretching.

What if I have existing health conditions?

It's vital to prioritize your health and consult your healthcare provider before embarking on a new exercise regimen, including yoga. Once you receive medical clearance, share your health concerns with your yoga instructor. A skilled instructor can adjust poses and sequences, ensuring a safe and nurturing practice that complements your medical needs.

By communicating openly with your instructor, you empower yourself to make informed choices that align with your well-being. The combination of medical expertise and yoga guidance creates a balanced approach that enhances your overall health.

I'm not anywhere close to being a flexible person, but can I still do yoga?

Flexibility is not a prerequisite for practicing yoga; it's a byproduct of consistent effort. Yoga meets you where you are, embracing your current range of motion. Gradually, through mindful practice, you'll experience an expansion of your flexibility and a newfound sense of comfort in your body.

Yoga is about self-discovery, self-acceptance, and progress that is unique to you. Your journey is marked by incremental improvements, fostering a deeper connection with your body and a sense of accomplishment with each milestone.

Will yoga help with joint pain?

Many seniors find relief from joint pain through a mindful yoga practice. Gentle movements and stretches promote joint mobility and alleviate stiffness. However, it's essential to approach your practice mindfully and attentively.

Yoga's holistic approach incorporates physical postures, breath work, and meditation, all of which contribute to your overall well-being. By engaging in yoga poses that support joint health, you can experience improved flexibility, reduced discomfort, and a greater sense of vitality.

Can yoga improve balance and stability?

Yes, yoga offers a plethora of poses that specifically target balance and stability. Engaging in poses like tree pose, warrior III, and chair pose strengthens the muscles responsible for balance while cultivating a greater sense of proprioception.

Through consistent practice, you'll notice improvements in your balance and stability, which can have a positive impact on your daily activities. Yoga's focus on alignment, breath, and mindfulness heightens your body awareness, contributing to enhanced overall stability.

Clearing up Misconceptions

Yoga is only for the young and flexible, not seniors.

This misconception couldn't be further from the truth. Yoga is a practice for individuals of all ages, backgrounds, and abilities. Senior practitioners bring a unique depth of life experience and wisdom to their practice, enriching their journey.

Yoga's inclusivity allows for the adaptation of poses and sequences to suit each practitioner's capabilities. By embracing your individual journey, you join a diverse community of individuals who are dedicated to well-being at any stage of life.

Yoga requires complex poses that seniors can't do.

Yoga is not a performance; it's a practice of connection. The practice encourages you to explore your body, embrace your limits, and nurture growth without comparison. Skilled instructors are adept at modifying poses, making them accessible while preserving their benefits.

Yoga's true essence lies in the journey of self-discovery and self-awareness. As you engage with poses that align with your abilities, you'll find that the practice becomes a celebration of your unique journey, free from expectations of perfection.

Yoga doesn't offer cardiovascular benefits for seniors.

While yoga may not match the intensity of some cardiovascular exercises, it still offers a range of benefits for heart health. Certain styles of yoga, such as Vinyasa or Power Yoga, incorporate dynamic movements that elevate heart rate and improve circulation.

Additionally, the emphasis on breath control in yoga supports lung health, enhancing oxygenation and promoting overall cardiovascular well-being. The practice's holistic nature nurtures your body's systems, contributing to your vitality.

I'm too old to start yoga now.

Age is not a barrier to beginning a yoga practice. In fact, many individuals discover the profound benefits of yoga later in life. Yoga supports senior practitioners by maintaining flexibility, balance, and mental clarity, fostering an enhanced quality of life.

Regardless of when you start, yoga's gentle and adaptable approach is designed to meet you where you are in your journey. Each pose, each breath, and each moment on the mat contributes to your well-being and growth.

Yoga won't help with mental health concerns.

Yoga's transformative power extends beyond the physical realm. Integrating mindfulness practices, breath work, and meditation into yoga can have a profound effect on mental health. These practices offer tools for stress management, anxiety reduction, and cultivating a sense of calm.

The practice of yoga encourages a mindful connection between your body and mind, promoting self-awareness and emotional balance. By embracing yoga's holistic approach, you embark on a journey that nurtures not only your physical well-being but also your mental and emotional wellness.

Yoga is religious, and I don't want to compromise my beliefs.

While yoga has spiritual roots, the practice itself can be adapted to align with individual beliefs and preferences. Many yoga classes focus solely on physical postures and breath, offering a secular and universal approach that respects diverse backgrounds.

If you're concerned about the spiritual aspect, seek out classes that emphasize the physical and mindfulness elements of yoga. This allows you to experience the numerous benefits of yoga without compromising your personal beliefs.

I need to be flexible to start yoga.

Flexibility is a journey, not a prerequisite. Yoga embraces your current capabilities and gradually enhances your flexibility over time. Each practice session contributes to your overall range of motion and comfort in your body.

Yoga's foundation lies in acceptance and self-discovery. By practicing with mindfulness and compassion, you'll find that flexibility is just one of the many benefits that unfold on your yoga journey.

Conclusion: Embracing Wellness Through Morning Yoga for Seniors

As we draw the final curtain on our journey through "Morning Yoga for Seniors," we stand at the intersection of wisdom and well-being, a place where age is not a limitation but a gateway to a more vibrant, balanced, and fulfilling life. Throughout this book, we've explored the remarkable potential of yoga to rejuvenate both body and mind, offering a tailored path for seniors to enhance their overall quality of life.

From the very first rays of the sun, as you embarked on your 10-minute morning yoga routine, to the profound moments of mindfulness and self-discovery on and off the mat, you've demonstrated the resilience and determination that define your journey. The benefits of morning yoga extend far beyond physical flexibility and strength; they encompass a deeper connection with your inner self and the world around you.

We've dismantled myths and misconceptions, acknowledging that age is not a barrier but a canvas upon which you paint your unique expression of yoga. Flexibility is a journey, progress is a tapestry woven through practice, and mindfulness is the cornerstone of well-being.

The journey of a senior practitioner is one of empowerment and self-nurturing. By embracing modified poses that respect your body's abilities, harnessing the power of breath, and delving into the richness of mindfulness, you've cultivated a resilient mind-body connection that reverberates through each step of your life.

Remember that your yoga practice extends beyond the mat – it's a way of living that infuses mindfulness into each breath, each bite of food, and each interaction. By integrating yoga into your daily routine, attending senior yoga classes for guidance and community, and exploring the transformative experiences of yoga retreats, you've embarked on a lifelong journey of well-being and self-discovery.

As you close this book, consider it not an end but a new beginning. The wisdom you've gained, the practices you've cultivated, and the connections you've forged are the stepping stones to a future enriched by vitality, balance, and joy. The essence of yoga now resides within you, a wellspring of strength, serenity, and self-awareness that continues to shape each day.

May your mornings be infused with the gentle stretch of a pose, the rhythm of your breath, and the embrace of mindfulness. May your days be a testament to the harmony you've cultivated between your body and mind. And may your life be a living testament to the transformation that is possible when we nurture our well-being with intention and care.

From the sunrise to the sunset of your journey, may you find solace, inspiration, and fulfillment in the practice of morning yoga for seniors. The mat is your sanctuary, the poses are your companions, and the journey is your masterpiece. With each breath, step, and moment of presence, you embody the spirit of yoga and pave the way for a life illuminated by well-being, connection, and the boundless possibilities that await.

Namaste.

ATTRIBUTIONS

Cover design and other elements used in this book were sourced from Freepik.com.

Printed in Great Britain
by Amazon

37177479R00031